Translating Spirituality and Medicine in the Healing Professions

A Physician-Clergy Handbook

Glenda F. Hodges, PhD, JD, MDiv
and
Harold B. Betton, MD, PhD

authorHOUSE®

AuthorHouse™
1663 Liberty Drive
Bloomington, IN 47403
www.authorhouse.com
Phone: 1-800-839-8640

First published by AuthorHouse 3/29/2010

ISBN: 978-1-4520-0562-1 (e)
ISBN: 978-1-4520-0561-4 (sc)

Library of Congress Control Number: 2010904081

Printed in the United States of America
Bloomington, Indiana

This book is printed on acid-free paper.

Table of Contents

Dedication

To healthcare professionals and clergypersons everywhere who are responding to a higher calling. May God continue to bless the fruit of your labor.

Glenda F. Hodges

and

Harold B. Betton

Foreword

Rarely have I witnessed a project that has been pursued with the type of sincerity and passion as the work that has been undertaken by Drs. Hodges and Betton in their quest to illustrate the connection between spirituality and medicine. When I began my tenure as Chief Executive Officer at Howard University Hospital in August 2007, I had recently attended the Spirituality and Medicine Recognition Banquet held annually in April as part of the Spirituality and Medicine Seminar Series. I was thoroughly impressed with the event.

Having spent a career that spans more than 30 years in hospital administration, I had never witnessed such an occasion that brought together physicians, other healthcare professionals and members of the clergy to celebrate persons who were advancing the union of spirituality and medicine. Each year that I have attended this event, it has grown in attendees and developed in scientific inquiry. It is a "one of a kind" production that has not, in my experience, been duplicated.

There is much that we do not know about science and there is even more that we cannot explain about our faith. We often request that our physicians do all that they can to help us maintain optimum health; however, when we follow their prescribed instructions, we expect a favorable result. Unfortunately, that is not always the end of the story. When the physicians adhere to their learned standards of practice and we experience a bad outcome, we often turn to our faith. For those of us who are Christian in our theological persuasion, we appeal to Christ Jesus. We allow our faith to give us the peace that helps us manage and cope with whatever we encounter. Even when we do not know how our situations will conclude, our faith sustains us.

Dr. Hodges and Dr. Betton are unrelenting in their quest to explicate the union of faith and science. As Christian ministers, they are encouraged by their own beliefs and are utilizing the same to encourage others. I applaud their work and it is my hope that they will continue to explore new avenues that will motivate others to think critically about the union of mind, body and spirit. Their work has certainly been an inspiration to me!

Larry Warren,

President and CEO

Howard University Hospital

Washington, DC

Foreword

To practice a profession is both a privilege and a responsibility. Embracing and understanding such a privilege and responsibility are connected to the basic definition of a true profession. Webster defines a profession as "an occupation requiring considerable training and specialized study." Two of the most rigorous, respected and essential professions known to humankind are the professions of ministry and medicine. Each demonstrates a 'caring' and 'healing' component, characterized by practitioners committed to promoting the total health and well-being of all people.

While medicine and ministry have usually been recognized and practiced as separate and distinct fields of endeavor, their origins are inextricably intertwined. Dating back to the most ancient documentation of human existence, there has been a consciousness and awareness that human beings are more than flesh and blood, more than anatomy and more than physiology. Every recorded culture has embraced human life as being transcendent and therefore valued far above its simple organic and cellular composition.

Personhood transcends the simple combining of essential yet complex, organic systems that together form a functioning human organism. Self-awareness, personal consciousness, self-esteem, perception of life and whatever gives value and meaning to life, greatly impact health and well-being. This has been substantiated by one of the true Fathers of modern medicine, William Osloer, MD, author of "*The Faith That Heals*," published in the British Medical Journal in June, 1910.

Accordingly, genuine health and wholeness must embrace the components of personhood. Such components cannot be easily measured by the extraordinary tools afforded by science and medicine alone. In order to increase our understanding of this area, a 'bridge' must be erected that evidences mutual respect and cooperation while illuminating the complementary professions of spirituality and medicine.

The courage and commitment to 'bridge the gap' between spirituality and medicine have been superbly embraced by Drs. Glenda F. Hodges and Harold B. Betton in their first book, *Spirituality and Medicine: Can the Two Walk Together.* In this initial offering, they marked themselves as pioneers and daring explorers on a journey into the ever expanding 'universe' of holistic, compassionate and comprehensive healthcare. Now they have taken the next step of the journey by giving us a practical model in the application of these interrelated concepts and strategies in this insightful and informative handbook, *Translating Spirituality and Medicine in the Healing Professions*.

They have used their years of experience with the Howard University College of Medicine and Howard University Hospital's Seminar Series in Spirituality and Medicine and convened critical work groups comprised of persons who embrace the professions of ministry and medicine. This has served as the source material to harness the experience and observations of those persons of dual professions who have successfully combined spirituality and medicine in their worlds of work. The end product of these work groups is a handbook that addresses issues and contains strategies that support the work of those "in the field" who are committed to excellence in comprehensive and holistic care for all people.

The handbook offers real food for thought for those who are committed to caring for others, but struggles to define the 'limits' of care giving. It challenges whether there is primacy in being distinguished as a classical healthcare practitioner and/or one who is 'called' to the ministry. While there are genuine conflicts that sometime arise in distinguishing and understanding the two areas, what often occurs is an expanding awareness of medicine in its truest sense. As related to me by a wise professor of medicine as he shared his concern about the impersonal direction of some areas of modern medical practice, "medicine is not a job but a calling!" What is 'primary' is compassionate, comprehensive care, which demands the most rigorous and continued education of the practitioner in order to deliver such care.

Genuine caregivers must always respect spiritual diversity and the boundaries determined by the patients' perspective. There are a number of resources that are available for both the healthcare professional and the clergy. Some use of these resources is essential if effective application is to occur. However, the key ingredient for comprehensive care is the development of mutual respect and a combining of resources by both professions in order to integrate what each has to offer in order to benefit those for whom they both provide care.

The section on Avoiding Burnout is a first step in understanding the importance of the dual roles of healthcare practitioner and clergy and clearly demonstrates the need for further development in this area, especially in view of the personality and character traits of many who feel called to either ministry or medicine or both!

The sections on Engaging the Parishioner and Thinking Outside of the Box will prove invaluable to those committed to caring as well as to those who are recipients of holistic healthcare. These sections should provide the foundation for envisioning and producing community based applications that are culturally relevant and cost effective in raising the level and quality of holistic healthcare to those most at risk. Hopefully, this information will provoke those who make healthcare decisions to reconsider what true access to healthcare looks like.

The fact that this handbook is written by Christians, primarily for those who are Christian practitioners, does not restrict its broader usefulness by those persons of other faith perspectives. While most relevant and applicable to those of the Christian faith, the manual can be widely applied to all practitioners, in general. It must be recognized that a key tenet of holistic healthcare is the health, well-being and perspective of the patient and, as such, should always be the central objective of the practitioner.

As a practitioner of both fields, formally trained in the practice of medicine and a senior pastor and church leader for over thirty years, I have seen the power of spirituality (God) and medicine work hand-in-hand. I applaud the authors and all those responsible for contributing to this monograph, which does a great job in melding spirituality and medicine. While the possibility that one's religion or spirituality positively influences health and healing is now almost universally accepted, mutual respect, cooperation and understanding by practitioners of both professions is still lacking and remains controversial. This handbook should serve as a model to help us rethink our perspective of these critical, interrelated concepts and simultaneously benefit those that we serve by helping us find innovative ways to apply these concepts.

Bishop Horace E. Smith M.D.

Division of Hematology, Oncology and Transplant

Children's Memorial Hospital

Northwestern University

Feinberg School of Medicine

Chicago, Illinois

Senior Pastor, Apostolic Faith Church

Chicago, Illinois

Presiding Bishop

Pentecostal Assemblies of the World, Inc.

Preface

Our first book, *Spirituality and Medicine: Can the Two Walk Together*[1], was devoted to discussing the observation that led to the natural conclusion that regardless of differences in beliefs, values and attitudes, spirituality and medicine have always coexisted. This book, a logical progression from our first one, details testimonials and other related experiences that provide convincing explanations useful to clergy and physician practitioners in translating the coexistence of spirituality and medicine in the healing professions.

Although we are Christian in our theological persuasion, the anthropological observations suggest that we are not limited by our theological orientation. We have con-

---

[1] Glenda F. Hodges and Harold B. Betton, *Spirituality and Medicine: Can the Two Walk Together* (Author House: 2009).

cluded that we are mere voices in the cultural outcry for health promotion and disease prevention and unrelenting ambassadors promoting the belief that God's power is supremely responsible for ultimate wellbeing.

We are particularly pleased that the annual Howard University Hospital's Spirituality and Medicine Seminar Series are continuing; our first book was an outgrowth of the first ten years of those seminars. However, as we have proceeded to enlarge our understanding in this area, we have begun to realize the need to translate our theories into practice. On June 5, 2009, we hosted a Physician/Clergy Summit where we brought together eleven professionals who were both physician and clergy. Our expressed goal was to discover a realistic and useful avenue in order to disseminate information to patients and parishioners with whom these professionals regularly interacted. At the culmination of our time together, we concluded that a Physician/Clergy Handbook would be a practical resource to accomplish this task. Additionally, we believed that this manual would be useful on a day-to-day basis to assist both physicians and clergypersons as they provided care to persons seeking both physical and spiritual guidance. To the best of our knowledge, this is the first pocket manual to be published with such an objective.

Inasmuch as we are Christians, we have chosen to write this manual for Christian practitioners. A manual written for the other major faiths would require more than an academic knowledge; it would also require an awareness predicated by practicing and living the faith. The physicians/clergypersons who attended our Summit are all confessed Christians practicing their respective professions and living their faith. Collectively, we affirm that Jesus Christ is the Son of God and it is through the Son that we (practitioners) are able to access the Father, constantly petitioning His guidance in the work that we do.

We are grateful for the support of Howard University Hospital's CEO, Mr. Larry Warren and his sincere commitment to advancing the union of spirituality and medicine. We also acknowledge the dedicated staff of the Division of Community Relations at Howard University Hospital. Most importantly, we are inspired by the Summit attendees who traveled from various places to add valuable input to this manual. They include the following persons: Reverend Dr. Anthony L. Mitchell, MD, Emergency Room Specialist and Minister, Macedonia Baptist Church, Bryans Road, Maryland; Reverend Kenneth S. Robinson, MD, former Shelby County, TN Health Commissioner and Pastor, St. Andrews African Methodist Episcopal (AME) Church, Memphis, TN; Reverend Lucille C. Norville-Perez, MD, AME Minister and Director of the Cave Institute, Bethesda, MD; Reverend Floyd L. Atkins, Jr., DPM, Associate Minister, St. John Baptist Church, Houston, TX; Reverend A. Oveta Fuller, PhD, Pastor, Bethel African Methodist Episcopal Church, Adrain, Michigan and Microbiologist, The University of Michigan, Ann Arbor, MI; Reverend Therman E. Evans, MD, PhD, Pastor, New Life Christian Center, Inc., Linden, NJ; Reverend Miriam J. Burnett, MD, and President, Resource and Promotion of Health Alliance Inc., Fayetteville, GA; Reverend William A. Holley, DPM, Associate Pastor, St. John Baptist Church, Buffalo, NY and Reverend Mark J. Wade, MD, Associate Pastor, True Vine Christian Center, Fair Lawn, NJ. Our Summit Facilitators included Reverend Dr. Glenda F. Hodges, PhD, JD, MDiv, Director, Howard University Hospital, Division of Community Relations and Elder, Reid Temple AME Church, Glen Dale, MD and Reverend Dr. Harold B. Betton, MD, PhD, Principal Physician, Betton Clinic and Pastor, New Light Baptist Church, Little Rock, AK.

Introduction

Anthropological data suggests that in most cultures, the physician-priest or Shaman was one of the more important individuals in the community. The Shaman's responsibilities were not limited and/or affected by the patient's age, gender or malady. As theology and medicine continued to advance, there developed a great divide in the realm of faith and science, thereby separating the roles of priest and physician. One of the by-products of this divide was the shift in the faith/science paradigm and the significant growth of each area that helped in shaping its respective cultural impact. To this day, this paradigmatic shift is still realized.

Most peculiar to this shift is the fact that God has remained a part of this paradigm as is evidenced by His divine intervention in the presence of all types of diseases. Accordingly, the spirituality and health dualism has always existed. In increasing numbers, patients are sharing their religious beliefs with their health care professionals as part of their physician/patient relationship. More and more health-history questionnaires contain questions designed to glean religious information. Hospitals are acknowledging the same by increasing the diversity of their chaplaincy staff and nursing homes are welcoming clergypersons from various faiths to attend to the spiritual needs of their residents.

Surprisingly enough, a present day Shaman, of sorts, has arisen within the physician/patient relationship. Many physician practitioners are being called into the preaching ministry while simultaneously remaining active within their home churches teaching, preaching, conducting religious revivals and participating in foreign missions and healing rituals. It is important to note that for purposes of this manual, the terms clergyperson, pastor, preacher and minister are used interchangeably to describe those individuals who are embracing the spirituality and medicine connection. Unlike the Shamans of yesterday, these persons are also serving in such roles as academicians, research scientists and attorneys. Of the physicians attending the Summit, two were church pastors and three were associate ministers with their local congregations. In addition, one was an attorney and elder in her local congregation; one was a research scientist and pastor; one was a former public health official and physician; two were actively practicing podiatrists and associate pastors of their local congregations and one was a physician-administrator and pastor of a local congregation.

The diversity of representation was vast among this exceedingly small sample. Indeed if one amassed a list of persons called by God to serve in the ministry or pastoral profession while maintaining their healthcare roles, the task would be daunting at best. We only hosted a group of eleven; however, our outcomes were such that we were compelled to share them with others as exemplary indications of how spirituality and medicine are coexisting in the healing professions. This pocket manual does not explicate the scientific basis of the connection; that was the purpose of our first publication, (*Spirituality and Medicine: Can the Two Walk Together*). Alternatively, it augments the efficacy of utilizing spirituality and medicine as a resource when caring for persons who desire to be made whole. The manual is divided into four areas of concentration, each answering a key question and expanding upon that information as it is translated into application to persons on their paths to total wellness.

As we sought to present our material in a user friendly fashion, we concluded that it would be best to begin by discussing the validity, utility and applicability of its content. In *Chapter One*, we begin by answering the following question: *What information can be placed in a pocket manual to promote the validity of the spirituality and medicine dualism for clergypersons and medical practitioners?*

Chapter Two is devoted to the pastor or minister in his/her pastoral care ministry and explicates concrete issues, tools of the trade, relevant legal concerns and specific resources that are useful in the healing professions.

Chapter Three explains the practitioner burnout problem. It contains helpful information designed to maintain the physical and mental health of practitioners in the healing professions.

Chapter Four provides useful information regarding the role of the parishioner/patient in the spirituality and medicine paradigm. Since many churches have healthcare ministries called by a variety of names, this chapter offers useful information to any church seeking to start or enlarge its sphere of influence in this paradigm. We have supplemented each chapter with questions that we hope will assist the physician/clergy practitioner in caring for those whom they serve.

The discussion entitled, "Thinking outside of the box," provides information that highlights means by which some churches have managed community problems while enlarging their circle of influence in the spirituality and medicine paradigm. For purposes of reader efficiency, we have added a section entitled "Resources" in the final portion of the book. This section includes sample questionnaires, legal documents and Internet resources which practitioners may use when discussing several comprehensive healthcare issues with patients. In addition, several blank, lined pages are included for purposes of reader notes and other entries.

Chapter One

The Healthcare Practitioner and the Call to the Ministry:
Is One Primary Over the Other?

During our Summit meeting, one of the attendees observed the following all too often observation. "When God called me to the gospel ministry, He did not tell me to stop practicing medicine; He simply enlarged my sphere of service." This observation may extend to any and all walks of life. God often calls us in the midst of our secular professions to enter His prescribed work on a full-time basis. It is certainly not the scope of this manual to second guess God's intentions; rather, it is the purpose of this chapter to discuss the call as it operates within the secular profession. In doing so, we emphasize four key areas. The remainder of the chapter provides illustrative conversation which elucidates these pertinent areas.

1. Which is primary, the practice of medicine or the call to preach and/or minister?

2. How does the call to the ministry impact the practice of medicine?

3. How do patients embrace the dual nature of a physician-clergyperson?

4. How do parishioners engage the clergyperson who advocates holistic ministry?

Which is primary, the practice of medicine or the "call" to preach and/or minister?

The answer to this question depends upon one's response to several variables, including theological persuasion, the definition and content of the call and how one assigns value to the call. Before anyone fully embraces the call of God to undertake a particular assignment, the import of the call must be defined and clarified within the theological dictum in which the individual operates. The formal structure which may very well determine how the call is manifested must clearly prescribe some sort of validation if the call is to be sanctioned by an organized group. Alternatively, one may acknowledge the call, self-validate its authenticity and proceed to carry out its mandates. It is our belief that one's response to God's ministry, above and beyond that for which one is secularly trained, must be clearly examined vis-à-vis its added value to the service of God.

While at first glance this discussion may appear complex and abstract, we believe that it has significant cultural and theological implications. In the Jewish faith, the call begins with a sincere desire to be a messenger for God. This usually precedes the course of study for a Rabbi. In the Catholic faith, the call is similarly inspired. In each of these faiths, persons choose to enter into the clergy profession by desire and may not have experienced what is defined as a divine calling from God.[2] However, for most Christian faiths, the divine call from God is paramount before *ordination* (religious validation) is considered and as such, testimony must be offered as part of the ordination catechism.[3]

The Muslim faith differs in that the first order of religious leadership is characterized by leading prayer services. The Imam begins this hierarchy and acceleration/promotion is based upon demonstrated knowledge in the following order: the Shaikh, Fazilatol, Shaikh and Allamah.[4] In Buddhism, the path to becoming a Buddhist Monk is not initiated by a divine call, but rather a personal

---

[2] http://www.helium.com/items/223899.

[3] Personal experience of one of the authors, Harold Betton.

[4] http://en.wikipedia.org/wiki/Islam.

desire to enter into the service of the Buddhist path.[5] The progression then takes the path of education in Buddhist practices and finally becoming accepted and trained by an Elder in the Temple of one's choice. It should be apparent why the nature of the "call" is complex in most religions; however, those responding to it must simultaneously recognize the awesome task and importance of exercising that call. Accordingly, those medical practitioners who answer the call are uniquely faced with the same dilemma, which is primary, the call or the practice?

We have concluded that a call by God expands one's horizon beyond that for which one is secularly trained and/or hired. As practitioners in the healing professions under the leadership of the master physician Jesus Christ, those with whom we interact must always see Jesus

---

[5] How to Become a Monk or a Nun – Preparing for Ordination. http://www.fomt.org/IMI/Firstletter.asp

Christ manifested in us. The call to the ministry enlarges our territory[6] and as such, we are recipients of that divine grace which lends itself to attending to the special health-care needs of those assigned to our care. We are entrusted with the responsibility of holistic,[7] preventive and restorative care. Dr. Anthony Mitchell, emergency room physician, preacher of the Gospel and Summit attendee, stated it best. "Instead of coming to the emergency room, we should be coming to the prevention room. At the end of the day, the call is dual, not separate."

How does the call to ministry impact the practice of medicine?

Schools that train healthcare practitioners do a commendable job in preparing their graduates in the praxis of disease prevention and health promotion; however, they

---

[6] The Holy Bible, King James Version (KJV), 1Chronicles 4:10.

[7] The Holy Bible, KJV, John 5:6.

fall short in merging these areas. Seemingly, prevention falls in the domain of the primary care practitioners and health promotion in the realm of specialized care. For the holistic care practitioner, respective of praxis, the Christ centered aspect of care demands that both prevention and promotion/restoration are simultaneously delivered. Dr. Mark J. Wade, Summit attendee, Associate Pastor and Pediatrician, observed that within the realm of holistic healthcare, persons must be educated in order to provide comprehensive care. This paradigm becomes expanded to include the good news of Jesus Christ while providing the care that is a usually a result of one's scientific training. Dr. Wade suggested that the clergyperson-physician is obligated to continue this paradigm until the deathbed. According to Dr. Wade, "If one is on the deathbed, the clergyperson-physician is obligated to ensure that the unsaved has the Gospel delivered to him/her and the practitioner must do whatever is mandated by the Holy Spirit to enable the patient an opportunity to accept Jesus Christ." Dr. Wade commented, that "death is one thing, but an unrepentant soul is something else altogether!"

When the practitioner places his/her call as primary in every aspect of healthcare delivery, then the scope of medical practice is enlarged so as to follow the basic tenets of the medical profession while embracing the direction of the Holy Spirit. We genuinely believe that the Christ-centered practitioner will always deliver the care that is in the best interests of the patient. Jesus' approach as He encountered the man at the pool of Bethesda is exemplary, in this regard.[8]   While recognizing that the man had been plagued with an illness for a long period of time, Jesus offered him an opportunity to be freed from the disease and

---

[8] The Holy Bible, KJV, John, Chapter 5.

8

restored to holistic health. This is a commendable example that illustrates the merging of the two areas of disease prevention and restoration of health.

Recognizing that the call to ministry is primary means that our responsibility to the One who has called us lies beyond our secular employment. We have a responsibility to share Jesus Christ, the Word, the Way and the Truth and to use wisdom in that paradigm. We are not suggesting that one preaches to the patient or attempts to proselytize, but rather that one uses every available opportunity to proclaim the good news. Although we are not proselytes, we are healthcare practitioners who are capable of offering both medical and spiritual instruction.

We recognize that our task is not an easy one. One possible approach is to first get to know the person, not the disease. Similarly, we must provide the patient an opportunity to encounter us. The practitioner needs to demonstrate to the patient that caring is equally as important as curing in the treatment paradigm. Hence, being known as a preacher in this paradigm is somewhat advantageous because there is an implication of greater compassion capacity within the workplace. The preacher/pastor-physician should have a greater impetus to explore whatever is needed for the inclusion of holistic healthcare. In reality, we believe that this translates to greater love and acceptance of the person before he/she is viewed as a patient.

Finally, to accomplish holistic healthcare, the pastor/preacher-physician must define his/her practice as patient-centered. Everyone, including the patient, must understand this focus. The practitioner need not attempt to validate any lifestyle; God assigns validity. However, the pastor/preacher-healthcare practitioner must be able to answer the hard questions that are often associated with providing care. These questions may include queries such as why the disease, how long will I live, what happens when I die, just to name a few.

How do patients embrace the dual nature of a physician/clergyperson?

Do patients really engage the healthcare practitioner who is also a clergyperson? Should the preacher-healthcare practitioner announce his/her uniqueness? One measure of disclosure, in such instances, is for the patient to see the Christ within the practitioner. The patient needs to understand and fully endorse the resource that accompanies the practitioner who is medically trained and simultaneously led by the Holy Spirit in his/her delivery of care. In this paradigm, the patient is central and the Holy Spirit is free to aid in the restoration of wholeness. When this scenario is realized, the patient is able to appreciate the uniqueness of the practitioner and is more likely to accept the practitioner's advice as given to the patient as directed by the Holy

Spirit. This is important for the comprehensive health of God's people!

Another important aspect of the preacher-practitioner's praxis is the role of prayer. Under these circumstances, it becomes a natural part of the treatment plan. It has been our experience (especially in the African-American community) that very few people, Christian or non-Christian, refuse prayer. What they seemingly conclude is that they are receiving treatment from a caring practitioner and at the end of the day, that is all that matters! All too often, it is a moment of crisis that has invaded the patient's place and space and he/she is ready to hear from you and all the resources that you bring with you. These are the occasions where God allows the practitioner to introduce and acquaint the patient with Jesus Christ and His ability to heal every disease and/or situation. We believe that "God is able to do exceeding abundantly beyond all that we can ask or think, according to the power that works within us."[9] As part of the treatment plan, prayer should always be according to the will of God in that person's life; God's timing is paramount. When patients fully accept the dual role of preacher-practitioner and the power of prayer, healing abounds even when symptoms of illness remain.

How do parishioners embrace the physician-clergyperson who practices holistic ministry?

The Summit attendees concluded that a large number of parishioners willingly accept the dual nature of the pastor/preacher-healthcare professional. Without exception, the practice and teachings of these professionals are Christ-centered and reflect the Biblical mandates that anchor our relationships with Christ Jesus. It should be noted that one of the disciples and author of several of the New

---

[9] The Holy Bible, KJV, Ephesians 3:20.

Testament writings was a physician companion of the Apostle Paul, Dr. Luke.

For the preacher/healthcare practitioner, the definition of holistic healthcare is expanded beyond the traditional definition as espoused by alternative care practitioners. Holistic healthcare attends to the mind, body and soul. The traditional standard of care may offer quick solutions to complex issues; however, holistic solutions are more exhaustive and require more time and patient participation. The preacher-healthcare professional's aim is to get to the root cause of the patient's problem. Within this nuanced paradigm, the patient is free to consider mind, body and soul as they collectively contribute to comprehensive wellness.

Conclusion

We believe that a call from God to serve in any capacity requires obedience to the content of that call. It is not expected that every healthcare practitioner will embrace the preacher/physician paradigm and, accordingly, may even have challenges attempting to merge the two. However, for those of us that have been "called from darkness into the marvelous light," we are quite comfortable in allowing the Holy Spirit to lead us as we assist in providing care for God's people. Each practitioner must respond to the call as he/she is directed.

To that end, this resource is designed for those practitioners who are called by God to merge both the science and the faith in order to achieve holistic care. We also believe that the manual will be helpful to practitioners of healthcare who are not clergypersons. We make no representation that the audience for this manual should only be physician-preachers and/or physician pastors, or healthcare practitioner/preachers and/or healthcare practitioner pastors. The manual is written with the goal that it will reach all who embrace their healthcare praxis with Jesus Christ as a part of their team. We utilize the terms healthcare practitioner/clergyperson, healthcare practitioner/layperson and clergyperson/preacher/minister/pastor to cover the landscape of all of those answering God's call.

We believe that God's call will impact one's healthcare praxis and pastoral care ministry. The extent to which this occurs will most likely depend upon the nature of the call, the responsibilities as well as the gifts and graces God chooses to bestow upon the one He has called. While all healthcare practitioners will not utilize their call in the same manner, each one must share a similar knowledge base and have access to similar tools. In our first book, previously footnoted, we outlined the necessary knowledge base to create the appreciation for the union of spirituality and medicine. This manual should be used in tandem with the first publication in order to supplement the resources available to all persons who seek to provide holistic care.

Anthropological evidence testifies to the truth of Paul's message that God created man with the knowledge of His presence and involvement in the lives of His created persons; therefore, man's rejection of God is baseless.[10] The material culture of many civilizations provides this evidence through its iconography. Lastly, the folklore of most cultures features a Shaman (priest or holy man) whose role rests with the merger of the spiritual-medical-health paradigm. It is from these observations that a fundamental basis is created for an understanding of the dual nature of

---

[10] The Holy Bible, KJV, Romans 1:20.

17

the physician/clergyperson. These individuals are naturally inclined to seek direction from a higher power.

Research indicates that patients rarely ask questions of their healthcare practitioners regarding the practitioner's spirituality. On occasion, inquiry may be made by the patient regarding the physician's church affiliation; however, such information is hardly, if ever, viewed negatively. Moreover, physicians across the theological spectrum take care of patients whose backgrounds are equally as diverse. In such a melting pot, those called by God to provide care must be resolved to use all of the resources at their disposal to ensure that their contributions are pleasing in God's sight. Under these circumstances, patient acceptance of the physician/preacher practitioner is rarely a problem.

It has been our experience that Christian parishioners wholeheartedly accept the dualism; they liken it to a fulfillment and extension of the Christian doctrine. All of us are taught to fulfill God's will in our lives and execute the same in our praxis.[11] All too often, the Christian parishioner will suffer because he/she does not believe that the pastor/healthcare practitioner transfers the comprehensiveness of ministry to the local congregation. The church has not developed the types of avenues and/or programs designed to emphasize holistic care. Much attention might be devoted to caring for the spirit; however, the same programs fall short in discussing the impact of the mind and the soul in comprehensive healthcare. This manual devotes a separate chapter for this discussion entitled, "thinking outside of the box." This latter discussion will contain numerous anecdotal testimonies from pastor-physicians that managed problems existing in the neighborhoods in which

---

[11] The Holy Bible, KJV, Colossians 3:17, 23.

their churches were located, by utilizing the healthcare spirituality dualism.

Translating This Application

Which comes first, the practice or the call?

The following scenario illustrates how this information can be translated to patient care. Four real-life illustrations are provided; two are inpatient and two outpatients.

Scenario One: Obedience to a divine appointment with a terminally ill inpatient

I remember the day as if it was yesterday, although it was at least 15 years ago. At 4:00 am on Memorial Day, I was asleep when I felt a definite touch on the backside of my left shoulder. The touch immediately awakened me and I heard a voice that said, "get out of bed, go to the hospital and see Mrs. _____; her soul will be required of me today." The patient to whom the voice made reference was one for whom I had been providing care. She had been admitted to one of Little Rock, Arkansas' finest hospitals. I obeyed the voice; I arose, dressed and drove to the hospital. Upon arriving, I entered the elevator and attempted to push the button to the 10th floor to start making rounds. Once again, I was directed to not push that button but rather push the button for the 6th floor, the location of my terminally ill patient within the medical intensive care unit.

When the door opened, the patient's husband and daughter were outside of the room as though they had been awaiting my arrival. I greeted them and told them that I came to check on my patient and all of us went into the room. As a matter of course, I obtained her chart, although I knew that I would have no need of it on this particular day. I entered the room, placed the chart on the table, said a few words of greeting and proceeded to discuss death and dying and the beauty of uniting with the Lord. After the discussion, all of us held hands and had prayer. Upon completion I said parting greetings, finished hospital work and returned home. At 1:00 pm, the same day, I received a page from the medical intensive care unit and I returned the call. I was informed that my patient had expired.

Which is primary, the practice or the call? In this example, the **call to minister** was certainly primary. There are times in the ministry when one is called to do out-of-the-ordinary things. For me as a physician, it is not unexpected to be required to weave this responsibility into the praxis of medicine. The patient and family had no idea of the extreme urgency and importance of that particular hospital visit on that day. For them, it was not really necessary; for me, it was expedient to respond to the divine call to ministry that I had answered years previously and to be obedient to the instructions that had been made clear to me by the One to whom I had responded. I know and recognize the voice of the Lord. He guides me in my practice in all that I do. When He speaks to me, I must obey. The renowned brain surgeon, Dr. Keith Black has said that "religion is a discipline that one pursues with passion; medicine is a passion that one pursues with discipline." His statement provides a wonderful analogy of the "call" and the "practice." Which comes first? We believe that when the question has to be answered by the practitioner, he/she will choose the right response!

Scenario Two: Direct intervention in diagnosis and treatment

In my practice, one of the more troublesome problems to treat is unraveling the diagnosis and directing the appropriate treatment when I have encountered a diagnosis classified as *fever of unknown origin*. Such was the case twenty years ago when I admitted an elderly, elegant, retired farmer and large landowner to the hospital. He had no unusual medical history or contact with infections. He had not experienced any recent travel. This person was being seen by at least four different consultants in addition to me and every conceivable option was addressed.

24

The medical care that he received was second to none, not because of who he was but because it was the right thing to do. Despite all efforts, his chart of temperature reflected that he would either leave the hospital with fever or succumb for lack of a diagnosis.

This particular day of rounds would be different. It was Sunday morning and I was at his bedside. I told him that I knew precisely who knew what was going on with his body and that his situation could be fixed. I asked him if he, like I, believed that the supreme physician, Jesus Christ, could fix anything. He voiced his belief in agreement. We held hands and I simply prayed that God would direct the physicians who were providing care to him on the correct path to fix *his* problem and restore him. On Monday morning, approximately 24 hours from the Sunday visit, I went to his room. His chart reflected that within less than two hours from my visit, his temperature curve returned to normal and he had remained free of fever. I observed him 24 more hours and he had no return of fever. He was discharged from the hospital. I took care of this fine gentleman an additional 10-12 years before his death at the age of 88. During this entire time, he never had another fever from any cause, not even a common cold.

Which is primary, the practice or the call? In this case each was equally important. Again, it was necessary for me to be obedient to the call. However, it was the intervention through the call that directed the practice. What is impossible for man is possible with God. It has been said that man's extremity is God's opportunity. All of my colleagues who were assisting me in providing care to this patient were baffled regarding the genesis of his fever. Collectively, we discussed the patient; however, none of us had the medical knowledge to proffer a treatment plan that would change the situation. In obedience to the Holy Spirit, I consulted the greatest physician, Jesus Christ. In this particular situation, He guided me in such a way as to utilize the medical praxis to cause the patient's fever to abate. I share this story to encourage other physicians and health-care professionals. It is no secret what God can do; what He has done for me in my practice; He will also do for you.

Scenario Three: Prayer for a worried mother

All of us have encountered the mother whose troublesome child has given her many sleepless nights. In this instance, the child was a wayward one, strung out on drugs and his mother had no knowledge of his whereabouts. My patient, the mother, was a very friendly person and we often engaged in conversation about her children, particularly this child. He had been in and out of trouble and on and off the streets. Despite this mother's prayers, tears and worry, the child never seemed to "hear her."

On the occasion of this routine office visit, the mother presented tearfully, worried that her child may be dead. She had not heard from him in weeks and she knew that he was in another state, most likely living on the streets and involved in some sort of drug behavior. After much conversation with her, we both concluded that the only person that could help her was God. During this particular office visit, we prayed, in the name of Jesus Christ, that her son would be found, arrested and placed in jail, prompting the necessary phone call to her.

In less than two weeks from that prayer the young man was indeed found, arrested and subsequently convicted of a nonviolent crime. He spent the necessary time in a penal institution and upon his release, was paroled into his mother's care. She brought him to the office where I had a chance to meet him and tell him the story. To this day, he is not the same person. The change that we witnessed in him was extremely positive and most phenomenal.

Which comes first the practice or the call? Obedience to the Holy Spirit's direction is always primary in the manner in which I care for patients. I believe that my ability to practice medicine is informed by my call to the ministry. While I never thrust prayer upon a patient, I am constantly seeking God's direction for his/her care. In this situation, I did not force prayer; I simply told her that I knew someone who knew the exact location of her son. When she asked me who it was, I explained that it was God. I then asked if she wanted to join me in prayer as we petitioned God for His assistance in locating her son. She immediately consented and we prayed together to the one "that is able to do exceeding abundantly beyond all that we can ask or think." God answered our prayer and the worried mother's condition changed. Long after her son came to live with her, she would continue to talk about the power of prayer and God's ability to heal her broken heart and spirit.

Scenario Four: Patient initiated prayer

As a family physician of 31 years, I have had many occasions to provide spiritual support to patients; however, this one is most illustrative of the spirituality paradigm. Many adolescents often get into trouble and, as juvenile offenders, may be brought in from the detention facility to my office for treatment if they are personal patients of my practice. Such was the case three years ago. A 14-year-old boy came in for treatment of his asthma. Upon beginning the examination, in my customary manner I extended my hand and received a handshake. I then proceeded to obtain his medical history, perform an examination, prescribe the appropriate medication and explain how it was to be administered. While I was not led by the Holy Spirit to do any more than this, the young man obviously felt that something else was necessary. Without any notice, he looked me in the eyes and said, "Dr. Betton, would you pray for me?" I immediately told him yes, put his chart down, invited the deputy sheriff to petition God with us and all of us joined hands in prayer for his welfare, safety and spiritual growth with the Lord Jesus Christ. In all of my years of medical practice, I had never had an adolescent to ask for prayer in the office. Without a doubt, I was very thankful to have been used as an instrument of God to provide spiritual support to this young man.

Which comes first the practice or the call? In this situation, I had provided the care as dictated by my medical knowledge. Because of the patient's request for me to petition God on his behalf, I prayed. Spirituality and medicine combined in such a way as to engender the comprehensive care that this patient sought. As a preacher-physician, one must remain open to the Holy Spirit and always willing and ready to respond to divine directives, regardless of whether initiated by the physician or the patient.

Remember...

1. The physician-preacher must remain open to hear the voice of the Lord as he/she cares for the patient. As such, God's voice is always primary.

2. The physician-preacher must recognize that just as God directs the medical praxis, God likewise paves the way for His will to be done.

3. The physician-preacher must understand the needs of the patient and family and ensure that those needs are always paramount.

Chapter Two

Resources Available to the
Pastoral Care Professional and the Healthcare
Practitioner-Clergyperson

A seminary education is designed to prepare students for the clergy profession just as a medical education prepares the healthcare practitioner to care for patients. Historically, each profession has reaped the benefits of several well prepared clergypersons and healthcare practitioners who are making a difference in comprehensive healthcare. However, several questions germane to our discussion merit consideration. It should be noted that healthcare practitioners and pastoral care professionals must have access to certain "tools of the trade" that help to enlarge their sphere of influence as they broach areas such as death and dying and end-of-life care. In this chapter, we have identified specific questions that grew out of our 2009

Clergy Summit that we feel are useful for healthcare practitioners and pastoral care professionals who are continually working together to unite spirituality and medicine.

Much controversy abounds regarding the current healthcare legislative debate and end-of-life discussions. Some senators have argued that one should not wait until the end-of-life to initiate the discussion; however, others feel that such a conversation is not relevant until the individual reaches the age of Medicare. For purposes of this manual, we have compiled several tools that are useful whenever the end-of-life discussion becomes important. These tools are introduced here vis-à-vis a list of questions that characterize the thinking of both preachers and physicians.

In what ways can pastors further holistic care beyond the generic hospital visits in medical settings?

In the first chapter of the manual, we covered the concept of preventing healthcare problems. Part of this prevention strategy should embrace the inclusion of the pastoral care professional. In this regard, we view no separation between the secular and the sacred and, as such, any resource that can assist in promoting comprehensive and holistic care should be made available to all practitioners. Everything begins with the recognition that human beings are mind, body and spirit. From that point, the conversation may easily move to the congregation, church and the faith community.

In the church environment, the pastoral care professional can easily introduce the notion of comprehensive wellness and aid in the understanding of the importance of the mind, body and spirit connection. Much of what is said and/or done in this environment moves into the home. If healthcare is emphasized in the home, it then moves to the community-at-large. In this manner, the pastoral care professional is viewed as a necessary link in the healthcare paradigm and offers significant insight well beyond the generic hospital visits that are routinely made as part of the clergy's responsibilities.

Traditional Sunday School still remains the backbone of most pre-Sunday worship service activities. This "school environment" provides yet another opportunity to emphasize healthcare. Creative pastoral care professionals may develop curricula that emphasize proper eating habits, exercise, life skills, health and wellness practices and workshops on living wills and financial preparations. These subjects can be easily woven into the Sunday School curriculum without causing disruption in the normal course of traditional instruction material.

Additional church-based programs such as "Kids for Education," tutorial classes, Report Card Review sessions and small group counseling are all viable approaches that may introduce an interconnectedness of mind, body

36

and spirit geared specifically to church youth. The back-to-school rally concept and the annual youth conferences are all part of the menu of services especially designed for youth and young adults. Such programs which emphasize the value of these young people to the church at large send a powerful message to them that should be harnessed and fine tuned for information on health promotion.

For the mature members of the congregation, as well as the young mothers and fathers, a culinary ministry that focuses on nutritional content of foods, their impact on health and well-being, dietary modifications and consequences, are all important and timely. Many young mothers do not cook full balanced meals on a daily basis, and as such, "quick-fire" cooking education is needed. Mothers and fathers need to know how to prepare nutritious meals in 30 minutes or less and they need to know the value of teaching toddlers proper eating behaviors so that these behaviors can be instilled in them as they grow older.

Many churches offer congregation wide fellowship meals and banquets; however, there is hardly ever a nutritional content discussion prior to the meal. The meal selection items do not detail nutritional content. Accordingly, this ministry can offer valuable insight into food preparation. For your health, proper eating habits may help to control glucose maintenance for diabetics, carbohydrate counting for control of diabetes, hypertension monitoring by consumption of leafy green vegetables and problems with hydration by focusing on the importance of water consumption.

Workshops on end-of-life preparation are also necessary. The audience at these workshops will usually vary. Persons who are in need of hospice care, those diagnosed with a terminal illness, as well as extremely healthy persons, are all excellent candidates for discussions on advance care planning. Specific topics may include living wills, healthcare proxy, power of attorney for healthcare, as well as estate planning. Internet sources on advance directives, tools that have been successfully used by others and sample planning documents may be distributed at these workshops. Persons leave these workshops empowered to make their wishes known regarding end-of-life care.

At the end of the day, trained congregants become trained patients and are able to interact with their physicians or healthcare practitioners on a different level. They become better equipped to handle changes in their lives and have a congregational-based resource to continue the discussion beyond the healthcare practitioner's examination room. Under these circumstances, the **church has become an extension of the prevention room**. It also becomes a living atmosphere in which the truth of John 5:6 is illuminated. One can easily discern the benefit of Jesus' question to the man that had lain by the pool for 38 years. The same question can be asked today, "Will you be made whole?"

How does standard seminary education equip ministers who utilize the spirituality and medicine connection?

The curriculum of most seminaries is fraught with theology, biblical studies and pastoral care courses. Little value has been given to the spirituality and health connection. We believe that purposeful training in this area is extremely important.

There are several avenues available in seminary education for the natural inclusion of this discussion. Senior seminar courses that include, as part of their component, an internship in pastoral care, linked with the hospital chaplaincy, are fertile ground for the spirituality and medicine connection.

We believe that hospital chaplaincy persons, as well as pastoral care professionals, realize the correlation between spirituality and health. In addition, a relevant part of their education occurs on-the-job, in prayer sessions with others and in life's lessons. Oftentimes, some pastoral care professionals embrace the union of spirituality and medicine by direct experiences, whereas others remain tenuous and unsure of the connection.

Educational efforts in this area need to be supported by the seminary education and seriously reviewed as facts, rather than nuances or anecdotes. We offer our first book, *Spirituality and Medicine: Can the Two Walk Together,* as a viable starting point for seminary educators.

To this end, it is currently being utilized as the principal text in the Bachelors degree program in Religious Studies in one of our nation's historically Black Colleges and Universities. In this course, the students are taught that no separation exists between the sacred and the secular and, students are encouraged to wholly integrate the study of body, mind and spirit. When clergy educators omit this pivotal area, they compromise the necessary information that unfolds the miraculous ministry of Jesus Christ.

What resources are useful to ministers and physicians in caring for the terminally ill or chronically ill parishioner or patient?

Accessible resource information is extremely important for the pastoral care professional. It is also important for all those persons who represent the landscape of physician-preacher. Generally, continuing education, local seminars or special training courses can offer this information; however, the busy lives of those in the healing professions are often characterized by hectic schedules and consummate fatigue. Accordingly, they miss valuable training opportunities.

Our research has indicated that many clergy professionals need further training in hospice and end-of-life care. They need to know how to assist families in identifying hospice care, gaining access to homecare assistants and home healthcare aids. While the information presented in this manual is not exhaustive, it does provide the comprehensive points necessary to help the practitioner launch the end-of-life discussions.

Advance Directive

This term is used generally to refer to oral and written instructions about one's future medical care in the event that one becomes unable to speak for himself. Each state regulates the use of its advance directives. There are two types of advance directives: a living will and a medical power of attorney.

A **living will** is a type of advance directive in which an individual places in writing his wishes regarding medical treatment, should he become unable to communicate at the end of life. The state law in which the will is executed may define when the will goes into effect and may limit the treatment to which it applies. An individual's right to accept and refuse treatment is protected by constitutional and common law.

A **medical power of attorney** is a document that enables an individual to appoint someone to make decisions about his medical care if he is unable to make those decisions. It may also be called a *healthcare proxy* or *appointment of a health care agent.* In many states, the person appointed is authorized to speak for the individual at any time he is unable to make his own medical decisions, not only at the end of life.

Generally, advance directives are designed to give an individual a voice in decisions about medical care if he becomes unconscious or too ill to communicate. So long as one is able to express his own decisions, the advance directive is not used and medical treatment can be accepted or refused. If, however, one becomes terminally ill and looses the ability to participate in discussions about his own treatment, then an advance directive is used, if it is available.

Both federal and state laws govern the use of advance directives. The federal law, the Patient Self-Determination Act, requires health care facilities that receive Medicaid and Medicare funds to inform patients of their rights to execute advance directives. All 50 states and the District of Columbia have laws recognizing the use of advance directives.

One such nonprofit organization, Compassion and Choices, provides free state-specific advance directive packages that may be mailed to interested individuals. These packages are provided for a nominal cost and are useful to individuals and their families in answering questions regarding advance directives. Since 1967, this organization has pioneered living wills and has distributed more than 100 million advance directives. Additionally, it monitors legislative changes nationwide and updates all state documents accordingly. There are a number of areas that may be addressed in an advance directive. Our next topic of discussion provides useful insight into one of these important areas.

Withdrawal of or Withholding Medical Treatment

An individual has a constitutional right to request the withdrawal or withholding of medical treatment, even if doing so will result in the individual's death. Honoring one's right to refuse medical treatment, especially at the end of life, is the most widely practiced and widely accepted right to die policy in our society.[12] Most medical, legal and ethical authorities agree that no ethical distinction exists between an individual's request to have life-

---

[12] Questions and Answers: Advance Directives and End-of-Life Decisions. Choice in Dying Publication, 1997.

sustaining treatment removed after it has begun and a request to withhold this treatment. The United States Supreme Court affirmed the constitutionality of honoring a refusal of treatment in the case of Nancy Cruzan in 1990. In 1997, the United States Supreme Court reaffirmed this right in its decision in the <u>Washington v. Glucksberg</u> and <u>Vacco v. Quill</u> cases and distinguished between these types of end-of-life decisions and physician-assisted suicide.

An individual's right to refuse treatment is still valid when he or she becomes incompetent. All fifty states and the District of Columbia authorize the use of a written advance medical directive to help honor the decisions of those who are not able to speak for themselves but who have recorded their wishes in an appropriate legal document. The living will and the medical power of attorney are examples of these documents. We have provided a discussion of both of these tools in the following section.

Living Will and Medical Power of Attorney

Generally the advance directive document contains the contents of the living will and the medical power of attorney. A definition of each legal designation is provided.

Living Will – a type of advance planning document that determines the end-of-life care that one should receive in the event he/she is unable to make this decision.

Medical Power of Attorney – a document that enables an individual to appoint someone to make decisions about his medical care in the event that he becomes unable to make these decisions. It may also be called a *healthcare proxy* or *appointment of a healthcare agent.*

A generic example of such an advance, specific to Arkansas State Law, is found in the section entitled Resources. It is written as a living will for a husband, although the gender language is interchangeable.

Home healthcare and community resources

It should be understood that the clergyperson is not the social worker and should not be strapped with the responsibility of obtaining these resources. While the clergyperson may be able to determine when the family needs help, he should not be placed in the position of having to locate and identify this help. The first step in obtaining needed resources for the patient is through the patient's physician. Family members are encouraged to pursue this discussion with the patient's physician, inasmuch as the physician's signature is required on all documents for insurance payment to the agencies.

In cases where durable medical equipment (wheelchairs, walkers, etc.) is needed, the family members are likewise encouraged to speak with the treating physician. If the patient is in the hospital setting and these things are needed before discharge, or at least in the home upon discharge, the clergyperson can encourage the hospital social worker to talk with the family about these needs and/or the family may be placed in contact with the hospital social worker. Generally, the social worker will carry the petition through to its completion.

We have found *medicare.gov* to be an excellent website for persons desiring to obtain a more complete discussion of Medicare benefits. Furthermore, encouraging the family to contact the patient's insurance carrier with specific requests is always appropriate. Many insurance companies have nurses assigned to beneficiaries and they help them through the healthcare system to obtain everything from needed services to transportation; they are typically called **case coordinators**.

Physician resources

"The primary role of the physician is to ask the questions, become aware of the issues and mobilize the resources necessary to address them."[13] We present the fol-

lowing examples of spiritual questionnaires that have been

shown to be beneficial in the delivery of comprehensive

care.

The first questionnaire is the **Index of Core Spiri-

tual Experiences (INSPIRIT)**. This questionnaire pos-

sesses a strong degree of internal reliability and validity. It

is useful in clarifying the existential reality of one's spiri-

tuality as opposed to mere adherence to rituals and doc-

trines.[14] G. McCord, et. al. developed the second question-

naire designed as a spiritual inventory that can be included

in any patient's record.

---

[13] Ibid.

[14] Jared D. Kass, et al., "Health Outcomes and a New Index of
Spiritual Experience," *Journal for the Scientific Study of Religion*
30 (1991):203-211.

This questionnaire uncovers much about the patient's spiritual nature and belief system.[15] It has been proven to be a useful tool in instances where more detailed information is necessary concerning the patient's spirituality. Other useful tools include The **Maugan's SPIRITual History**, **HOPE Questionnaire** and the **American College of Physicians' Questionnaire**.[16]

Collectively, these tools are helpful when attempting to identify the spiritual beliefs of the patient. Additionally, the tools are invaluable in promoting continuity of care when evaluating the patient's progress. Under these circumstances, the utility of these tools may be likened to a situation where one would obtain a hemoglobin A1C for

---

[15] G. McCord, V. J. Gilchrist, S. D. Grossman, et al. "Discussing Spirituality with Patients: A Rational and Ethical Approach."

[16] Harold G. Koenig, *Spirituality in Patient Care: Why, How, When, and What* (Philadelphia: Templeton Foundation Press, 2002).

diabetic control, blood pressure for hypertension control or a blood urea nitrogen or creatinine for renal stability. By necessity, the tool must be quick and easy and administered at some predetermined or regular interval, commensurate with the patient's clinical status.

Unfortunately, the aforementioned spirituality questionnaires, which are often used in medical settings, are not very functional when following patients over a sustained period of time. They fall short in revealing changes in the patient's spirituality in the continuity of care paradigm. Further, testing an appropriate tool would require extensive research in varied settings.

In the absence of a validated tool, many physicians have opted to avoid questions regarding the patient's spirituality and only emphasize in the questionnaire the patient's health history. In these circumstances, we have determined that the spirituality of the patient is a crucial component in his/her health history and should be memorialized accordingly. As such, the Betton Spiritual Inventory and Continuity of Care Model are offered as components to include in the health history questionnaire. These tools are found in the section entitled Resources.

Life and death decisions are often a preoccupation of those that are terminally ill. In this regard, it is necessary to spend some time assessing these issues because they are paramount to the quality of life of the patient. How can one ease the pain of a terminal illness? What legal issues are relevant and how can the legal community be of assistance? The following discussion is intended to elucidate these issues. Many people have an awareness or understanding of heaven or some sort of afterlife, but are not prepared for the journey. Hopefully, this information will explicate those issues associated with end-of-life decision-making.

One source, as previously mentioned, for identifying useful tools for the healthcare professional, is the Internet. A search engine that we highly recommend is Google. New websites on the horizon are continuing to offer up to date and more helpful information. For a listing of these websites, consult the section entitled, Resources.

Clergy Resources

As clergypersons, we recognize that there is a body of information at the fingertips of most pastoral care professionals that will provide much of the information that we are intending to convey. However, this information is contained in several sources. We are bringing the greater majority of that information together in one manual that is user friendly for any healthcare professional. Additionally, we propose a sample form that we believe to be useful in providing after-hospital-care of the acutely or chronically ill parishioner. This tool is also found in the Resources section of the manual.

We recommend that this form be placed on file for future care that might be needed by the patient. The file should be shredded when it is no longer needed. We suggest that a new form be completed for every inpatient encounter, updated at least semiannually for every nursing home resident and at least once during each hospice admission. It is our belief that adherence to these recommendations will reduce the probability of Health Information Privacy Portability Act violations.

***What occasions, if any, are appropriate for hospice refer-
ral discussions with terminally ill parishioners?***

If the pastoral care professional assigned to the local congregation remains abreast of the parishioners' needs, hospice care discussions become easier. Remember, congregationally based workshops are always appropriate occasions to introduce relevant information in the healthcare arena.

Translating This Application

Spiritual Resources in Patient Care

Regardless of the unique medical specialty of the physician-preacher, knowledge of a patient's view of spirituality is important. The outcome of many procedures is linked to the patient's faith, not only in Jesus Christ, but also in whomever is placed in the patient's path for help. Many physicians recognize the faith-outcome link and welcome the help of clergypersons and other spiritually based resource persons as part of the patient's interdisciplinary healthcare team. Consider the following two illustrations.

Scenario One: When all seem to lose hope, faith must prevail.

Ms. L. is a young 52-year-old woman, the mother of several fine children, avid church attendee and president of her church's missionary society. All was well until this vibrant woman suffered a severe infection landing her into the intensive care unit of a local hospital. As her pastor, I knew quite well about her faith in the Lord Jesus Christ and her desire to continue to serve Him.

Visiting her on her second hospital day, she had a "code blue" right in front of me and cardiopulmonary resuscitation began immediately. Within less than 15 seconds of the resuscitative efforts, a physician friend of mine, a cardiothoracic surgeon, was walking toward her bed when I told him to promptly take over. My pastoral needs were urgent. Since her daughter and I were in the room when she "coded," I knew that the family was in disarray. After visiting with them and praying for them, I received a phone call that she had coded again. Fortunately, she survived all of the cardiovascular drama. Some physicians thought that she would not survive and had apprised the family of this possibility.

Ms. L. was not the kind of woman that would have accepted such a prognosis. Her chart clearly indicated her belief in spiritual and health matters, that she prayed regularly and that her physician should use spiritual counseling whenever and wherever appropriate for her or on her behalf.[17] At this time, as her pastor and physician, I entered into her record that she was to be afforded every lifesaving intervention short of nothing. All measures were taken, the necessary consultants remained and the end of the story is that she survived. We are pleased to report that she attends church every Sunday and uses every available opportunity to give the testimony of how God spared her life.

Sometimes the healthcare team may withhold certain interventions if the family decides to withdraw acute care in lieu of supportive (non-resuscitative) care. In this particular case, the medical history of the patient illustrated

---

[17] Betton Spiritual Inventory (Permission for this testimony has been obtained from this patient, though her identity in this publication is withheld).

the potential for the level of care that I knew she and her family wanted and expected. Without this information in the chart, the treating physician could have easily made another determination.

Translating spiritual knowledge into patient care is an important intervention because the healthcare team's actions can be modified by such knowledge. Careful consideration should be given to the following points as the healthcare team provides holistic care.

1. It is important to ensure that the outpatient record contains a document that succinctly addresses the patient's spirituality.

2. The healthcare team should gather as much knowledge as possible concerning the patient's spirituality because such knowledge may affect actions and interventions.

3. Periodically, the physician professional and/or other members of the healthcare team should revisit the spirituality area with the patient and chart whatever changes are discovered.

Chapter Three
Avoiding Burnout

Both the physician-preacher and the clergy professional can experience professional burnout. A number of questions come to mind when burnout is associated with persons in the healing professions. What causes this problem? Why is it so prevalent among physician and clergy healers? How can it be reduced and/or avoided? Is there special training that might be helpful in this area? Lastly, are there best practices that might be learned from pastoral care professionals that might be useful to medical professionals? These are only a few of the questions that we will tackle in this chapter.

Causes of Burnout

Dedication to one's professional responsibilities does not necessarily have to lead to burnout; however, when a false balance exists between professional and personal time, burnout can often be the ultimate result. Professionals who find themselves in this paradigm generally suffer from the same problem -- a sense of urgency (*right now*) to do what they have defined as God's will! Very often this leads to a one-sided lifestyle, strained family relationships and personally abusive behavior. The clergyperson (albeit physician or professional clergyperson, pastor, or pastoral care minister) rationalizes this behavior by asserting that God's work is preeminent to everything else. The family initially accepts this idea; however, when one too many important things are missed or one too many family members are disappointed, confusion erupts and things quickly go from bad to worse. The busy clergyperson walks a "tight rope" while juggling everyone's needs at the exclusion of his or her own needs. Sooner or later "hands are thrown up" and the downward spiral of burnout begins.

We believe that the scenario previously described can have a different ending. Prayer and meditation are generally part of the professional's life; however, he/she rarely takes time off to just be a spouse, family member or even take a vacation. Individuals that fall victim to burnout have difficulty setting limits and boundaries. They often enable their own burdensome lives by saying "yes" to most requests and almost never saying "no."

Avoiding burnout requires the ability to set reasonable limits. Physician and clergy training rarely present guidance in this area. We offer the following strategies as possible burnout prevention techniques.

1. Schedule a minimum of two vacations annually that are not centered on a professional activity.

2. Make it a point to spend quality time with your family and meaningful time with your spouse or significant other.

3. Consider a professional sabbatical and consult organizations such as the Lilly Foundation for possible funding of the same.

4. Seek continuing education courses that discuss topics relating to burnout that also offer prevention strategies.

5. Build an active exercise regimen into your daily life. Physiologically, the production of endorphins during exercise causes a feeling of wellbeing, which alleviates feelings of despondency. In addition, exercise improves cardiovascular health and stamina.

6. If you are a bi-vocational clergyperson, make sure that the two are not clashing or competing with each other.

7. If the professional is experiencing more serious problems, do not be afraid or reluctant to pursue qualified, professional counseling.

Quite often, pastoral care training allows for introspective reflection and discernment, which provides space for God to give much needed direction. Learn to "let go and let God." Know and recognize God's voice in your life. Be prepared to alter your personal plans to conform to His ultimate will for your life. It is amazing the sense of relief that can be enjoyed when you become the "passenger" and leave the "driving" to God!

It is important to distinguish pastoral care training from seminary training. Pastoral care training often teaches and prepares the minister to work in institutions where healthcare delivery is more intense. As such, setting boundaries and reserving judgment are the hallmarks of ensuring that ministry does not contribute to your overall state of becoming unwell. It is extremely important to allow all of the educational training to appropriately interface with the work that God has called you to do. While a number of ministry tasks may actually be learned by "on the job train-

ing," it is nonetheless important to use your professionally

acquired skills to help you stay on the right course.

In some instances, the pastoral care professional

may be residency trained. He/she may sit for the appropri-

ate licensing examination in counseling. In such instances,

the pastoral care professional usually has a Master's level

divinity degree (MDiv) with CPE units. These CPE units

represent a method of learning that strengthens pastoral

competence while the professional serves as a chaplain to

persons with a multitude of crises in a variety of settings.

We distinguish between the two professionals to offer the

following best practices.

Translating This Application

1. Attend pastoral care ministry conferences in your city and/or get to know a hospital chaplain who is residency trained in pastoral care ministry.

2. Obtain a current listing of conferences offered by the National Association of Pastoral Care Counselors (https://aapc.org/content/article-ii).

3. If interested in the vocation, become certified in pastoral care. The certification process can be found at the following web address: https://aapc.org/webfm_send/114 or http://www.aaiddreligion.org/certification/pastoral-care.

4. In order to join the National Association of Pastoral Counselors, visit https://aapc.org/content/article-ii.

5. Participate in support groups: Many ministerial alliance and local pastoral care organizations have

regular meetings. Often discussions with colleagues can help to identify beginning stages of burnout. Peer-to-peer discussion and fellowship is therapeutic and may be helpful in avoiding burnout altogether.

6. Become a member of an organization that addresses the union of spirituality and medicine. The National Medical Association (NMA) meeting has included a discussion of spirituality and medicine as part of its yearly convention content. Take the opportunity to become familiar with this material and use it in your respective profession. Invite presenters of this content material to your local parishes to enlighten other clergy colleagues who might also be experiencing similar challenges.

Chapter Four

The Health-Faith Paradigm:
Engaging the Parishioner

It is crucial that the role of the parishioner in the health-faith paradigm be explicated. Failing to do so would be tantamount to an egregious act. While we recognize that this statement is particularly strong, we do not want to miss the opportunity to convey the seriousness of the parishioner's role. After all, it is the parishioner that becomes our best advocate and probably our most vocal spokesperson when faith in God yields a desired outcome. Accordingly, it is the purpose of this chapter to build the bridge for the parishioner connection and to discuss strategies for its implementation.

African American churches have traditionally had its hands in health related issues regarding parishioners. The Missionary Circles, Nurses Guilds and associated

71

splinter groups were the original home health agency persons and community health-watch groups for the Church. The Nurses Guild took care of members at all Church gatherings, whether they were inside the physical building or attending outside church functions. In some instances, parishioners consulted members of the Nurses Guild even *before* they consulted their physicians. These organizations were viewed as legitimate and vital to the Church and its mission.

How are we managing health related issues in the church today? What is the complexion of health in the 21st century church? Does the church have a voice when disease is being discussed and/or when a health pandemic occurs?

Persons attending our 2009 Physician/Clergy Summit concluded that crisis, chronicity and cure represent the three focal points facing parishioners when disease is discussed. Similarly, these issues may also be recognized in a number of churches because the church is usually without a plan to address global health concerns. Several questions become relevant: What modules are useful in teaching health-faith principles to our parishioners? In what ways can the parishioner become part of the spirituality and medicine team? Lastly, what should be the components of a spirituality and health curriculum for the local church?

Rather than manage health issues in the church by the crisis intervention approach, identifying several portals of entry can serve as a useful mechanism to help those in need of health related services. These portals include support groups, sick and shut-in lists, prayer teams, first response units and numerous other options which are useful in matching the needs of the parishioner with the appropriate health-related service.

In the realm of holistic healthcare, the church becomes a key member of the team within the African American community. Within the church, the faith-health paradigm reaches its zenith in the realm of faith. However, the pastoral professional must stay focused on reality (signs, symptoms, and definition of disease) and how that reality interfaces with appropriate treatment, including faith and medical intervention. We offer the following six components which are useful when the church begins to fully engage its health ministry:

1. Educators,

2. Mentors,

3. Navigators,

4. Health Advocates,

5. Health Promotion Volunteers (HPVs) and

6. Support Group Leaders.

In the realm of education, a discussion regarding the etymology of the disease is always a good place to begin. Such topics as Biblical mandates and models, prophecy, generational impact and intent of disease should also be raised. Scripture is replete with wonderful examples that enhance the education area. Once this discussion begins, it is very likely that additional questions may evolve. This provides an excellent occasion to introduce support groups. They may very well tackle issues surrounding the following questions:

1. Why do I have this illness?

2. Is my illness connected to sin?

3. Am I being punished?

4. Am I going to die?

Please note that it is not the mission of the support group to provide concrete answers for these questions; but rather to create an opportunity where such conversations can occur.

In the process, it is hoped that the group can discover truths that will provide whatever the members need to deal with the issues surrounding their illnesses.

Mentors are always viable resources when change is introduced within an environment. The church is ripe with persons who are willing to support the cause of health education. Many of these persons are employed in health-related fields; others have personal testimonies of healings that have become part of their conversations with others. It is important to engage as many persons as possible to move the parishioners toward an understanding and acceptance of the spirituality and medicine connection.

Navigators are useful in directing persons into municipal outreach settings where they are able to access the healthcare delivery system. Mentors serve in capacities of both prevention and support. Within this group, HPVs may also be helpful in teaching more responsible healthcare practices in order to promote health and prevent disease.

How does one start a healthcare ministry within the local congregation? The first requirement is to identify a health and wellness team consisting of the following:

1. Volunteers,

2. Peer Partners,

3. Health Promotion Advocates,

4. Champions,

5. Service Providers,

6. Legislative Fundraising Persons,

7. Coordinators, Researchers, Evaluators and Data Collectors.

The extent to which certain team members are needed will vary based on factors such as congregation size, ages of members, church location, etc.

Churches may use various ways to delegate the mission of creating a Health Ministry. Some may choose to enlarge the roles of present ministries such as the Missionary Society or the Nurses' Guild, while others might make a general appeal to the congregation to determine interest and support. Whatever methodology is used, the end result should be toward building congregational support for health promotion and disease prevention. The Health Ministry should, at some point, become integrated into the other ministries of the church and become a viable resource for helping parishioners access the healthcare system. In the next section, we have provided strategies that should be considered to help the ministry "get off the ground."

Translating This Application

1. Survey your congregation and determine the prevalence of illness; this is accomplished by a simple health-related questionnaire that omits demographic information. (We have included one that might be useful.)

2. Meet with key church officials and create an automatic "buy-in" for the ministry.

3. Identify a member of the church that works well with others and is capable of advancing new initiatives and offer that person the leadership role in the ministry. (The person need not be a healthcare worker.)

4. If several Associate Ministers serve in your congregation, the pastor may choose to organizationally place this ministry under his/her supervision, as opposed to one of the other Associates.

We suggest a healthcare survey be done within the congregation and the results of the survey be used to tailor the health ministry to the specific needs of your congregation.

Thinking Outside of the Box

By virtue of the fact that many churches face new challenges across the membership and community perspective, instances will arise when ministry will interface with and confront various problems that face the church. Such was the situation encountered by Dr. Therman Evans, Pastor of New Life Christian Center in Linden, New Jersey. We have included his experience as an example of an approach that may be modeled, where appropriate, in other communities.

Adjacent to the present church building that New Life Christian Center occupies was an apartment building situated in what is described as "the number one crime ridden area of the city." The church purchased the building, renovated it and supplied affordable, very decent housing to the neighborhood. According to Pastor Evans, there usually exists a lengthy waiting list for occupancy of the units. As a result of the efforts of Pastor Evans and his members, the Mayor and Police Chief of Linden recognized New Life Christian Center for single-handedly reducing crime in the community in which the church is located. This simple, yet bold, economic act improved the community, added to the safety of the church members and improved the lives of God's people. Rather than turn their back and throw up their hands, they acted collectively. We include this as an illustrative example of thinking outside of the box.

The second intervention led by the New Life Christian Center was a community walk designed to reduce crime in the community. In this venture, men of the church numbering in excess of 150, walked the community twice weekly and talked with people, encouraged them, invited them to worship services and maintained a steady presence in the community. This intervention made it difficult for the criminal behavior, which had formerly plagued the community, to continue. As a result, crime dropped and more community stability resulted. This simple intervention exceeded the expectations of the church and the community-at-large.

Many communities are in need of spiritual Centers of Excellence, apart from the local church. Our youth are challenged and stretched beyond measure to find appropriate role models and behavior that they can emulate. Spiritual centers that concentrate on removing health disparities and increasing healthcare accessibility are extremely necessary. These centers usually emerge from church centered healthcare ministries.

We have identified a Center in Little Rock, Arkansas that is worthy of note. The pastor of a local Methodist church developed a need based ministry over 20 years ago and it has since become one of Little Rock's major philanthropic outreach centers. This center specializes in job training and procurement, feeding the hungry, housing the homeless and intervening in the lives of persons whose lives have seemingly spiraled downward. This spiritually based center of excellence's reputation is heralded across the state for its effectiveness in addressing the needs of those who are without. The Center provides assistance for persons across the demographic, socio-economic spectrum.

Another center of excellence that often exists within many communities is the healthcare clinic. This community resource specializes in addressing the healthcare needs of the uninsured and under-insured. Many of these clinics also grew out of religious organizations and have ultimately maintained a connection to some faith based institution.

Thinking outside of the box ministries represent those initiatives that arise from need based issues, whether they are interventions on behalf of a person, population, or a community. It is our belief that these centers are living examples of the great commission that is found in Matthew 28:19. This is evangelism at its best!

Epilogue

As previously mentioned, this manual is distinguishable from our first publication, (*Spirituality and Medicine: Can the Two Walk Together.*) We provide this writing as a user friendly guide for persons in the healing professions who are interested in furthering the spirituality and medicine connection. Whether physician, scientist, healthcare professional or full-time clergyperson, this manual adds value to the ministry to which you are called. An introduction of the science without strategies for implementation does a disservice to those of us wishing to advance the spirituality and medicine paradigm to the next level.

This manual was divided into four chapters, each providing a unique contribution in this paradigm and each providing strategies that enable implementation of its content. It is conceivable that all chapters will be germane to everyone and for that reason, this pocket compendium is designed to have universal appeal. Certainly this book does not exhaust all concepts that might be raised regarding translating spirituality and medicine in the healing professions; however, it does begin the conversation and provide the fabric upon which others may build.

The Howard University Hospital remains committed to advancing the spirituality and medicine conversation. Accordingly, it is our intention to continue the annual Seminar Series. Our hope is that many will join in the mission designed to connect faith and science. We are convinced that we are sowing into fertile soil and we remain encouraged to share our work with all who pursue holistic healthcare.

Resources

Sample Living Will Declaration
and Durable Power of Attorney for Healthcare of
xxxxxxxxxxxxxxxx

I, _____, being of sound mind, having reached the age of eighteen (18) years, residing in the State of Arkansas, do hereby make, publish and declare the following:

Article I

Living Will Declaration

(a) **Declaration**. If the time comes when I can no longer take part in healthcare decisions for my own future, let this statement stand as an expression of my wishes and my declaration while I am of sound mind:

(1) *Incurable or Irreversible Condition.* If I should have an incurable or irreversible condition that will cause my death within a relatively short time with no reasonable expectation of recovery, and I am no longer able to make

decisions regarding my medical treatment, I direct my attending physician, pursuant to the Arkansas Rights of the Terminally Ill or Permanently Unconscious Act of 1987, to withhold or withdraw treatment that only prolongs the process of dying and is not necessary to my comfort or to alleviate pain.

(2) *Permanently Unconscious.* If I should become permanently unconscious, I direct my attending physician, pursuant to the Arkansas Rights of the Terminally Ill or Permanently Unconscious Act of 1987, to withhold or withdraw life-sustaining treatments that are no longer necessary to my comfort or to alleviate pain.

(3) *Life-Sustaining Treatments Withheld.* These life-sustaining treatments which may be withheld or withdrawn include, but are not limited to: ANTIBIOTICS, ARTIFICIALLY ADMINISTERED NUTRITION, ARTIFICIALLY ADMINISTERED HYDRATION, CARDIAC RESUSCITATION, RESPIRATORY SUPPORT, AND

SURGERY. Notwithstanding any state law to the contrary, I hereby claim my constitutional right protected under the Fourteenth Amendment, as expressed by the United States Supreme Court in the case of *Cruzan vs. Missouri*, to refuse the artificial delivery of food and fluids.

(b) **HealthCare Proxy**. Should my attending physician have any questions or matters requiring interpretation with regard to this declaration, I direct my attending physician to follow the instructions of my wife, _____, whom I appoint as my HealthCare Proxy to decide what life-sustaining treatments should be withheld or withdrawn. In the event my wife, _____, should be unable or unwilling to serve or continue serving as my HealthCare Proxy, for any reason, I then appoint _____ as my HealthCare Proxy.

Article II

Power of Attorney for Healthcare

(a) **Nomination of Agent; Powers of Agent**.   During any period in which I am incapacitated, in the opinion of my attending physician, or am unable to make or communicate a choice regarding a particular health care decision, I hereby delegate health care decision-making powers to my wife, _____, as my Agent to exercise the authority described below relating to matters involving my health and medical care from time to time or at any time in my Agent's sole and absolute discretion. In exercising the authority granted to my Agent herein, my Agent should try to discuss with me the specifics of any proposed decision regarding my medical care and treatment if I am able to communicate.   Pursuant to the foregoing, and to the extent allowed by law (including Act 1448 of the 1999 Arkansas General Assembly), my Agent is authorized as follows:

91

(1) *Power of Access and Disclosure of Medical Records and Other Personal Information and HIPAA Release Authority.* To request, receive and review any information, verbal or written, regarding my personal affairs or my physical or mental healing, including medical and hospital records, and to execute any releases or other documents that may be required in order to obtain such information, and to disclose such information to such persons, organizations, firms or corporations as my Agent shall deem appropriate.

I intend for my agent to be treated as I would be with respect to my rights regarding the use and disclosure of my individually identifiable health information or other medical records. This release authority applies to any information governed by the Health Insurance Portability and Accountability Act of 1996 (aka HIPAA), 42 USC 1320d and 45 CFR 160-164. I authorize any physician, healthcare professional, dentist, health plan, hospital, clinic, laboratory, pharmacy or other covered healthcare provider, any insurance company and the Medical Information Bureau, Inc. or other healthcare clearinghouse that has provided treatment or services to me or that has paid for or is seeking payment from me for such services to give, disclose and release to my Agent, without restriction, all of my individually identifiable health information and medical records regarding any past, present or future medical or mental health condition, to include all information relating to the diagnosis and treatment of HIV/AIDS, sexually transmitted diseases, mental illness and drug or alcohol abuse.

The authority given my Agent shall supersede any prior agreement that I may have made with my health care providers to restrict access to or disclosure of my individually identifiable health information. The authority given my Agent has no expiration date and shall expire only in the event that I revoke the authority in writing and deliver it to my healthcare provider.

(2) *Power to Employ and Discharge Health Care Personnel.* To employ and discharge medical personnel including physicians, psychiatrists, dentists, nurses, and therapists as my Agent shall deem necessary for my physical, mental and emotional well-being, and to pay them, or any of them, reasonable compensation.

(3) *Power to Give or Withhold Consent to Medical Treatment.* To give consent to any medical procedures, tests or treatments, including surgery; to arrange for my hospitalization, convalescent care, hospice or home care; to summon paramedics or other emergency medical personnel and seek emergency treatment for me, as my Agent shall deem appropriate; and under circumstances in which my Agent determines that certain medical procedures, tests or treatments are no longer of any benefit to me

or, based on instructions previously given by me are not desired by me regardless of benefit, to revoke, withdraw, modify or change consent to such procedures, tests and treatments, as well as hospitalization, convalescent care, hospice or home care which I or my Agent may have previously allowed or consented to or which may have been implied due to emergency conditions.

(4) *Power to Contract.* To contract on my behalf for any health care related service or facility on my behalf, without my agent incurring personal financial liability for such contracts,

(5) *Power to Protect My Right of Privacy.* To exercise my right of privacy to make decisions regarding my medical treatment and my right to be left alone even though the exercise of my right might hasten my death or be against conventional medical service,

(6) *Power to Authorize Relief from Pain.* To

consent to and arrange for the administration of pain-relieving drugs of any kind, or other surgical or medical procedures calculated to relieve my pain even though their use may lead to permanent physical damage, addiction or even hasten the moment of (but not intentionally cause) my death; to authorize, consent to and arrange for unconventional pain relief therapies which my Agent believes may be helpful to me, and

(7) *Power to Grant Releases.* To grant, in conjunction with any instructions given under this Article, releases to hospital staff, physicians, nurses and other medical and hospital administrative personnel who act in reliance on instructions given by my Agent or who render written opinions to my Agent in connection with any matter described in this Article from all liability for damages suffered or to be suffered by me; to sign documents titled or purporting to be a "Refusal to Permit Treatment" and

"Leaving Hospital Against Medical Advice" as well as any necessary waivers of or releases from liability required by any hospital or physician to implement my wishes regarding medical treatment or non-treatment.

(b) **<u>Durability</u>**. This power of attorney is intended to be a Durable Power of Attorney for Health Care, in accordance with Act 1448 of the 1999 Arkansas General Assembly, and shall not be affected by my subsequent disability or incapacity.

(c) **<u>Successor Agent</u>**. In the event my wife, _____, is unable or unwilling to serve as my Agent for the purposes contemplated hereunder, then _____ shall serve in such capacity.

EXECUTED this _____ day of _____, 20__.

ATTESTATION

_____, in our presence voluntarily signed this instrument. Before he signed it, he declared to us that the foregoing instrument was his Living Will Declaration and Durable Power of Attorney for Healthcare and requested that we act as attesting witnesses to its execution. We now, in his presence and in the presence of each other, execute our signatures hereto as attesting witnesses to the foregoing instrument this _____ day of _____, 20__.

Name

_____

Acknowledgement

State of Arkansas

County of _____

BE IT REMEMBERED, that on this day came before me, the undersigned, a Notary Public within and for the County aforesaid, duly commissioned and acting, _____, to me well known as the person in the foregoing instrument of writing, and stated that he had executed the same for the consideration and purposes therein mentioned and set forth.

WITNESS my hand and seal as such Notary Public on this

_____ day of _____ , 20___.

Notary Public

My Commission Expires:

_____

(SEAL)

Betton Spiritual Inventory

We believe that it is necessary to include in our manuscript an unbiased spiritual inventory. In this regard, we offer the Betton Spiritual Inventory which has been used with much success in Dr. Betton's very busy outpatient practice.

Spiritual Inventory Questions:

1. Do you believe that spiritual and health matters may be related? Yes_____No_____

2. Do you believe that your doctor should use or refer you for spiritual counseling when appropriate? Yes_____No_____

3. Do you spend personal time in prayer or meditation? Yes_____No_____

Stress Inventory Questions

1. Would you describe your life as stressful? Yes_____No_____

2. Do you handle stress well? Yes_____No_____

3. Have you ever sought help for stress or nervous-
ness? Yes_____No_____

If the patient responds "yes" to question two of the spiritual inventory, the practitioner has the green light to inquire appropriately and a green dot can be placed on the back of the chart. Conversely, a red dot identifies that patient who does not desire spiritual counseling.

Within intervals set by the practitioner, the Betton inventory provides continual insight into the patient's illness from a spiritual perspective. This 6-question survey can be given as often as necessary in an effort to direct the practitioner to secure other services, such as chaplaincy, personal spiritual counseling, or other interventions which may stabilize or improve the patient's well being. Even if the person does not consider himself as spiritual, the research has indicated that serious or chronic illnesses may cause one to be more willing to discuss his/her personal spirituality. Repeated use of the Betton Spiritual Inventory by practitioners within the Betton Medical Clinic has yielded the conclusion that the document has consistent value in uncovering spiritual information about the patient.

For the continuity of care setting, Dr. Betton uses a six-point questionnaire designed to determine changes in the patient's spiritual and physical outlook. Similar to the Betton Spiritual Inventory, the questionnaire can be administered as often as necessary in an effort to identify shifts in one's spiritual outlook. It also provides information that is helpful in determining the need for acute spiritual interventions, either by the health care provider or the chaplain. We have included it in this manuscript to further explain its utility.

Betton Continuity of Care Model

This model is designed to evaluate the following 6 principal points about a patient.

1. An assessment of one's self in relation to being ill,

2. An assessment of care received and the providers of care,

3. An assessment of spiritual assurance,

4. An assessment of one's relationship with God or his/her higher power,

5. An assessment of one's assurance about his/her eternal outcome and

6. An assessment of illness burden.

Continuity of Care 6-Point Questionnaire

Instructions:

Rate on a scale of 1 to 5, where 1 is the lowest and 5 is the highest, your answers to the following questions. Circle your answers.

1. I feel good about myself and my outlook on life.

   1 2 3 4 5

2. I feel good about the care that I am being provided.

   1 2 3 4 5

3. My relationship with God or my higher power is continually strengthened.

   1 2 3 4 5

4. I cherish my quiet times for meditation or prayer.

   1 2 3 4 5

5. I am spiritually secure enough that I no longer worry about dying.

   1 2 3 4 5

6. Though I am aware that I have a serious or chronic

   illness, living with it is not a great burden.

   1   2   3   4   5

Advance Directive Internet Sources

1. http://www.oregon.gov/DCBS/SHIBA/docs/advanc e_directive_form.pdf (this site provides sample advance directive form that needs to be completed.

2. http://www.legalzoom.com/ (this site has a variety of legal forms available at no charge).

3. http://www.legalwriter.com (this site has forms for the medical power of attorney).

Clergy Post Hospital Tool

Name, Hospital, and Room Number:

_____

Contact name and phone number:

_____

Condition (stable, critical, ICU...)

_____

Family Information check list:

___Advance Directive inclusive of healthcare proxy, living will, medical power of attorney.

___Name of Primary Care Physician

___Permission to share any medical information with others including church (HIPAA complaint document on file)

___Hospital discharge date and other applicable information obtained.

___HIPAA complaint information signed on the reverse side of this card

Dates of scheduled procedures:

_____

Side B

HIPAA COMPLIANT DOCUMENT:

Patient Name:_____

Name of Healthcare proxy or Medical Power of Attorney:

_____

By my signature I,_____ (patient name or name of proxy/medical power of attorney) give my Pastor or his designee by name_____ permission to receive medical information from the following persons:

_____Patient   _____Healthcare proxy

_____Medical power of attorney

_____Attending Physicians

The information received is not to be shared with anyone unless it is cleared by one of the authorizing persons above. If anyone at church needs further information they are directed to call or contact: _____

_____

Signature and Date

Healthcare Survey Instructions

Your church is interested in creating a Healthcare Ministry, which would be responsive to your health needs and concerns. In order to do this, your feedback is needed so that the health education programs, provided by this ministry, will be useful in health promotion and disease prevention.

For each of the following questions, place an X in the space provided that best represents your response. Thank you for your cooperation.

Healthcare Survey

1. Do you presently suffer from any of the following ailments or diseases? (Check the ones that apply).

__diabetes   __high blood pressure

__cholesterol   __ heart disease

__HIV/AIDS   __sickle cell anemia   __obesity

__cancer   __other

2. If you suffer from any of the above, are you presently under the care of a physician? __yes __no

3. Are you presently taking any medications? __ yes __no

4. Have you ever been hospitalized for any reason? __yes __no

5. Do you receive annual "well-person" exams, such as pap smear, mammogram, prostate screening? __yes __no

6. Are you more than 30 pounds over your ideal body weight?

    __yes __ no

7. Are you involved in a regular exercise program? If yes, how many times a week? __yes __no

8. Have you ever been on a diet or been involved in a supervised weight-loss program? __ yes __no

9. Have you ever been diagnosed with a sexually transmitted disease? (STD) __ yes __ no

10. Are you presently sexually active? __ yes __ no

11. Do you use any form of birth control or contracep-tive? _____yes _____no

12. Have you ever visited a naturopathic (natural health care) doctor? _____yes _____no

13. Are you presently a caregiver? Do you care for a parent, relative, child or other person?

    _____yes _____no

14. Do you presently have active health insurance?

_____yes _____no

15. Do you feel that your overall health would be improved if your church had a Health Ministry?

_____yes _____no

16. Would you attend health education programs sponsored by the Health Ministry? _____yes _____no

17. Have you ever abused alcohol and/or drugs?

_____yes _____no

18. Would you like to be a member of the Health Ministry, if your church decides to create one?

__ yes __ no

19. If your church creates a Health Ministry, how often do you think it should meet?

__once a week   __once a month

__once a quarter   __as determined by the Pastor

20. List any programs and/or activities you would like

to see included in the Health Ministry.

Personal Notes

Made in the USA
Lexington, KY
06 June 2011